PASS YOUR PT TEST!

An Unconventional Guide to Passing the Air Force Physical Fitness Assessment

David Soto Jr.

David Soto Jr.

Copyright © 2016 David Soto Jr.

PREFACE

The content in this book is not intended to be a substitute for professional medical advice, diagnosis, or treatment. Always seek the advice of your physician or other qualified health provider with any questions you may have regarding a medical condition. Never disregard professional medical advice or delay in seeking it because of something you have read in this book. Blah blah blah.

I get a lot of advice about making sure I have citations and stuff, that way people would take me seriously but that seems not at all like the kind of book I like to write. Most of the content in this book is either real life experience or my opinion. I did do some research and state some facts in this book but did it in such a general way that I don't feel citations were needed. That's the kind of writer I am. I break stuff down to the point that anyone can understand it and leave it up to the reader to research the subject further on their own, if they want.

I feel I write for people who aren't prone to read medical studies, for people who want to just get to the good stuff without all the five-dollar words. I write this way because that's the kind of reader I am. People seem to like it. I was afraid that my first book, The Complete Guide to Primitive Eating, was too small and was lacking content but then the reviews started coming in. Turns out, the thing that I was afraid of was the very thing people praised the most.

I am not a professional by any means. I do not have a college education, unless you count my Associates Degree from the Community College of the Air Force in Mechanical and Electrical Technology, which most people don't. I am not certified in anything. Nor do I have any letters in front of or after my name, unless Jr. counts. I am just an average guy who has read a lot of books, done a lot of research, and conducted a lot of experiments on himself. My goal is to take all this information and put it in the hands of other average people out there like me, with hopes of helping them reach their goal.

I truly hope you enjoy this book.

David Soto Jr., Tucson, AZ

TESTIMONIALS

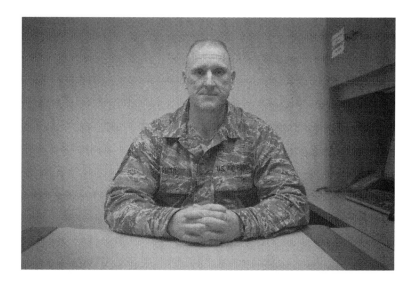

"I wanted to thank you personally for helping me pass the USAF physical fitness test. I had become complacent in my efforts to maintain fitness standards after 26 years in the military. In March of 2015, I only managed to attain a failing fitness score of 71.5. As a result, I was placed on the fitness improvement program of my unit. Thanks to your fitness and nutrition expertise, I was able to drop pounds and inches from my waist as well as improve my running technique that allows me to run without knee pain. When I re-tested four months later (July), not only did I pass the USAF PFT, I CRUSHED IT WITH AN EXCELLENT RATING of 92.3!"
~Eric Smith, SMSgt, MOANG, St. Louis, MO

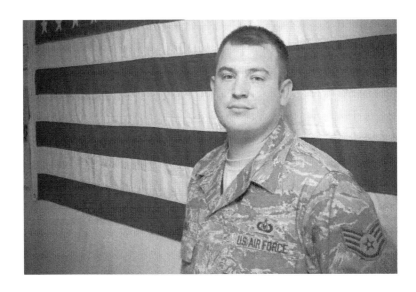

"I have suffered multiple (10) knee surgeries over the last decade. So I deal with chronic pain daily... on top of that my wife and I lost our youngest son in May. So I went into a deep depression and gained a bunch of weight. Without doing any training, I took my PT in early September. I measured at 38.5, 41 pushups and passed the walk. Ultimately I failed with a 73.3. Well, that fail was an eye opener for me and I felt the pressure with my MSgt Line # on the line. I began to research ways to lose weight and feel better, and that's when I really took a hard look at your program. With your program and coaching I lost 15lbs and 2.5 inches off my waist in 2 weeks. I am sleeping better, body doesn't hurt as bad every day. You have really helped me." ~J.R. Ford, TSgt, USAF, Tulsa, OK

INTRODUCTION

I retired from the Air Force and Missouri Air National Guard in December of 2015. I spent many of my last years not loving it and I'll be the first to admit, it had a negative effect on my life as well negatively impacting on my unit. Somewhere in the month of December 2014, I woke up one morning and realized I was going to be doing some things for the very last time in my life. For example, January's 2015 drill was the last Saturday and Sunday in January that I would ever wear the uniform. I had an entire year of events like this about take place, last annual training, last family day, etc.

Knowing all this, that I only had a year left in uniform, I wanted to make the biggest impact I could so I started writing Pass Your PT Test articles for my unit and coming in early to speak to those in the Fitness Improvement program. I have to say it was the best year of my career and I can honestly say that I loved every moment of it.

This book is the accumulation of those articles. In this book I'll break the PT test down into three sections: the run, the push-ups and sit-ups, and the waist measurement. The advice I'm going to give you is unconventional and unlike anything you have ever heard. Some of it may even be the exact opposite of what you have heard. But, if that information was working for you, you wouldn't be reading this.

PART ONE

AEROBIC ENDURANCE

RUNNING, FOOT & ANKLE MOBILITY

Typically there are two areas that make the run difficult: The pain we feel in our shins, calves, and feet, and the pain we feel in our lungs and chest. I'm going to give you three tips and action steps to take to help prevent the pain we get in our calves, shins, and feet during our run. Let's get to it.

1) **Squat** - And no, I do not mean 5 sets of 10 to make your behind nice and round. I mean, get into a deep squat and hold it for as long as you can. Then do it again and again and again. You might not even be able to get into a squat and if you can, it might suck. This is exactly why you need to do it. Squatting is one of the most natural positions your body is designed to be in. The problem is, you spend many hours of your day, for the majority of your life, training your body not to squat. If you doubt how natural it is, let me point out the first resting position a child takes after learning to stand. Also, in most of Asia, the deep squat is a comfortable position of rest as well as work.

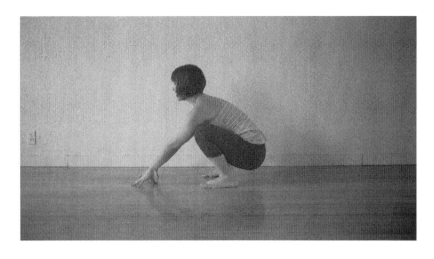

So why do it? It is the one movement I could give you that would work best to counter the years of damage sitting has done. There are a couple more I would suggest but I am trying to simplify here. Although squatting puts a load on all parts of your body, I am concerned with the load on your shins and calves. They are so tight that their range of motion is limited. You "program" these parts to sit at a 90 degree angle for hours at time every day. No wonder they hurt when you try to get them to move in a direction they are not used to (when you run).

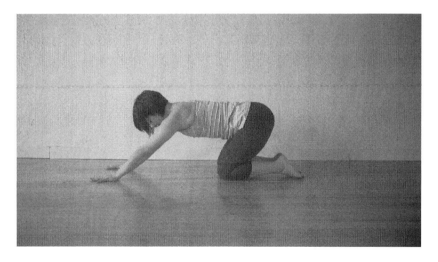

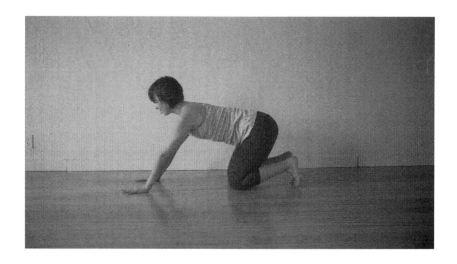

If you cannot handle the load of your body weight, squat without it. Do this by getting on your hands and knees and pushing your rear towards your heels. A bonus to this is you can do this in two positions. Toes tucked under or tops of feet flat, both are excellent for you. Get in these positions as much as possible throughout the day, EVERY DAY.

2) **Walk** - A lot. I mean, shoot for 20 miles a week. The treadmill doesn't count. This is a very natural thing for your body to do and it is so often neglected. Walking stimulates digestion and helps drain the lymphatic system, but more importantly, it gets your body used to doing something you want it to do in the PT test: Move forward!

I know you want to be able to run but you can't, at least not very well. Putting in miles upon miles of moving forward under your belt will train the very muscles and connective tissue you are going to use to run without the harshness of actually running. I promise, if you are used to walking 20 miles a week, running 1.5 is going to be a piece of cake.

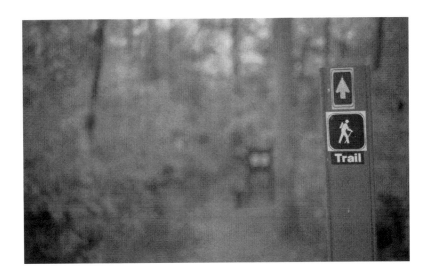

Want to really excel your progress? Walk on anything but flat smooth surfaces such as concrete and asphalt. Instead, hit the trails!

3) **Ditch the shoes** - You need to strengthen the muscles and connective tissue in your feet. "Support" may actually be damaging your feet by not allowing you to use the muscles as they were designed to be used. Shoes have been compared to wearing a cast. If you have ever had to wear a cast, you know that your muscles get atrophied and you have to build the strength back up after the muscles have been isolated for so long. Now imagine how weak your muscles would be from wearing a cast every day of your life.

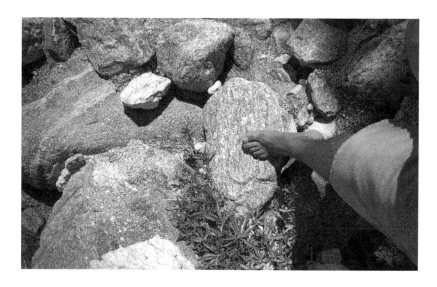

Do not go running barefoot! Although it is very beneficial, if you do not know what you are doing, you are going to get hurt. Instead, slowly introduce going barefoot. Try walking or doing your normal workout barefoot. Jumping jacks, jogging in place, or jumping rope for a few minutes a day are a good start.

If going barefoot seems just too "hippy" for you, at the very least get some "zero drop" minimalist shoes. They don't have to be those ugly toe shoes either. Anything without a raised heel will be better than what you are probably wearing right now. Even Chuck Taylors would be an improvement.

Ultimately, the key would be to get out of the boots you have to wear every day. Impossible right? I thought so too until I recently discovered Belleville Minimalist Boots. If you get these boots you will be working improving your run for eight hours a day without any extra effort. The difference in the heal height will help stretch your calves.

RUNNING, CARDIO VASCULAR ENDURANCE

Now, to address the pain in our chest, which is typically caused by our burning lungs. This pain comes from the demand your body has for oxygen. If you are experiencing this, it is because you are so sedentary that a little bit of exertion causes a high demand for oxygen. A lot of exertion will actually cause you to have to stop what you are doing. You know what I am talking about if you have ever been running and had to walk for a little bit to "catch your breath". If this is you, I hate to say it, but you are out of shape.

The good news is that we can fix this. Quite easily, in fact. What I want to address is how to train your heart and lungs without doing ridiculously long runs and how to decrease the demand for oxygen when you run (or, how to run efficiently.)

Sprints

These are going to suck, but the good news is you only have to do them for a few minutes a couple times a week. Better than going for a run, huh? There are many reasons and methods for this training. I have done a ton of research, but to save us both some time, I am going to give you one general method and reason.

Why do sprints? Simple. It is a way to target your heart and lungs without over-working and tiring your joints and muscles. Going for a five-mile run will work your heart and lungs very well, but can you run five miles? How about three? Even if you can, you're not only putting a lot of strain on your legs and feet, you're taking up a lot more time than you need. Besides, running 5 miles for leisure and 1.5 miles for time are two different things.

Action Step: Do 6 to 10 minutes of sprints twice a week. Get somewhere where you can flat-out run for 10-20 seconds. Running outside and barefoot is the best but do what you can. Get a stopwatch or use a timer app on your phone, and go! Run with everything you have for 10 seconds and then rest for 50. Do six rounds of these. Each round is equal to one minute. The two variables here are the amount to time you sprint and the amount of rounds you do. Use your best judgment and work at your own pace to get to the point where you are doing 10 rounds of 20 seconds on and 40 seconds off.

(Just a side note: Have you ever compared a sprinter's physique to a marathoner's?)

Run efficiently

Use less energy when you run and you will be able to run faster and farther. Makes sense, right? I was told once after a PT test that I "looked" like I ran slowly. I ran a sub 12:00 minute mile and a half. Not bad for this old man. Looking like I was running slowly can be attributed to running efficiently. I wasn't huffing and puffing, pumping my arms, bobbing up and down, swinging side to side or pushing off with my feet. Instead, I was running with relaxed bent arms, bent knees, landing on the balls of my feet and picking my knees up. Picking your knees up is the key.

The best way to do this is to stand up, bend both of your legs a bit, and jog in place, kind of like you are doing high knees only not too high. When you are jogging in place like this you will notice that your feet aren't going behind you but are instead staying in front of you. This is where you really see the efficiency. Because they are not behind you they can't push off the ground. When you are pushing off you are essentially doing a one legged calf raise. Do some of those now. Seriously! Single leg calf raise, go! Now, using that same leg, raise the knee up and down by bending it. Which of these could you do for a longer period of time?

Ok, once you have a relaxed, slightly high kneed jog-in-place going, it's time to actually start running. All you need to do in order to do this is lean forward at the ankles and away you go. The goal is to get 180 steps per minute. No more. This will help you stay efficient. Now, you may be slower when you start running this way but doing more steps per minute is not the solution. Leaning forward is. This is where that ankle mobility I talked about comes into play. The only thing that can slow you down running this way is lack of dorsiflexion (The ability to bend your foot towards you).

Action Step: Go for a run using the techniques I mentioned above, no matter how short (Not your sprints). If there is one thing I could tell you to remember when you are out there it is to **bend your knees.**

PART TWO

STRENGTH

GREASE THE GROOVE

Push-ups and sit-ups, believe it or not, are skills. This means they can be learned. If you want to learn something, you need instruction, but after that, you need PRACTICE! You need to practice every day.

This is where we run into problems with strength training. Through years and years of bad information, we have been associating strength with muscles. Big muscles mean super strong, right? So let's get big muscles! Let's lift heavily in gym, fatigue our muscles, get super sore for a few days, and then repeat the process a week later. Wrong! What we need to do is practice. Practice, practice, practice every day. But how can we practice when we are so sore we can't even take a sip of coffee without being in pain? Don't we need rest days and whatnot?

Let's take a look at how we would learn another skill, playing guitar. First you would get instruction: how to hold the guitar, how to strum, how to hold a pick. Then maybe some chords: G, D, E minor, F and C. Now that you have all this information you are ready to play Freebird, right? Wrong! What are you missing? How about hours and hours of practice. Why? Because you are not good at this skill. If you have ever played guitar, you know that one of the hardest things to do is change from one chord to another. Taking your finger from 5 locations and moving them to 5 different locations on the fret board is difficult at first. Do you think the reason you can't do this is because you are not strong enough, or does it have more to do with your brain and the signals that fire, telling you to put each of your fingers in a specific location? If you started practicing and did a Brian Adams and "played till your fingers bled," guess what you cannot do the following day or the day after that? You can't practice, the very

14

thing you need to do to get better. This is what is wrong with conventional strength training.

So let me sum everything up in one sentence: Do as many push-ups and sit-ups as you can every day, without getting sore. How do we do this? We "Grease the Groove."

Typically, "Greasing the Groove" involves doing a percentage of your max repetitions of a certain movement. Example: The max repetitions of push-ups till failure are 10. You do sets of 50% of your max throughout the day. This might look like 8 sets of 5 push-ups, totaling in 40 push-ups in that one day. Because you didn't go to failure and break down your muscles, you get do it again the very next day. Practice! Do this for 5 to 6 days a week and in a month re-test your max reps again. You should notice a significant difference. Did you get stronger? Yes, but you also trained your nervous system to treat this movement as second nature. This, in turn, requires less effort to accomplish the task, which gives you more energy to do more of them.

Another thing to keep in mind is that muscles aren't the only thing that make you strong. Connective tissue plays an important role too. Maybe more than actual muscles. Have you ever shook hands with someone who uses them for a living. Their strong grip does not come from finger curls. Nor do they have giant hand muscles.

Action step: Grease your push-up and sit-up groove.

Pavel Tsatsouline, the creator of "Grease the Groove", says if you want to get stronger, never do more than 5 repetitions of a movement. So, what I want you to do is one to five push-ups and sit-ups every hour on the hour, daily. Forget about your max. Start with one rep an hour. Take your total at the end of the day and try to beat it the next. If one rep feels like a piece of cake, bump it up to two the next day. Eventually you will be doing sets of five throughout the day. Do the best you can. Do not get fatigued! The key is to do as many as you can without breaking down your muscles and getting sore. At the end of your first month, you can progress on to doing a percentage of your max. Try for 30% to 50%. This may take you over the 5 rep restriction.

PART THREE

WAIST MEASUREMENT

REDUCING INFLAMMATION

I'll address losing weight in a couple chapters. This chapter and the next are about reducing the inflammation around your gut.

You have more than likely experienced acute inflammation when you sprained your ankle or got stung by a bee. The result is the affected area can become swollen, red, painful, or even warm. Typically these affects go away over a short period of time, when the threat is gone. If the inflammation persists, it is a good indication that something more serious is actually wrong. People who thought their wrist was sprained often find out it is actually broken after the swelling does not go away after a couple days

Chronic inflammation, which can be caused by consuming irritating foods, effects your body the same way as acute inflammation (pain, swelling, redness, and heat) but is present over a long duration of time, months or even YEARS. Imagine your body's reaction to a bee sting never going away. Now imagine this bee sting happening inside your body.

I want you to keep in mind that you heart and lungs are protected by your ribcage. They are also separated from the rest of your internal organs by a wall of muscle know as the diaphragm. Your diaphragm basically lies horizontally right at the bottom of your rib cage. Right below your diaphragm are your liver and stomach. Now if these two organs swell up due to inflammation, where do you think they are going to go? Not up. You diaphragm prevents that. How about down? Nope, your other organs take up the rest of the space in your thoracic cavity. The only option is OUT! This is the part of your belly you can't seem to get rid of and exactly where they measure waist for your PT test.

You may or may not have excess body fat but if you have a belly, especially right below your rib cage, I am willing to bet a big part of that is inflamed organs.

You can exercise and restrict your calories all you want but if you are still eating irritating foods, neither will reduce the inflammation in your gut. This is why, for a lot of people, diets don't work.

Below are just a few irritating and inflammatory foods:

1.   Wheat
2.   Sugar
3.   Dairy
4.   All Other Grains
5.   Booze

Action Step: Give up number one on the list above: wheat.

This includes all breads, tortillas, cereals, pancakes, waffles, pastas and sweets made with flour. Keep in mind, most things that are labeled "gluten free" are processed junk. They will likely still cause inflammation and definitely spike your insulin.

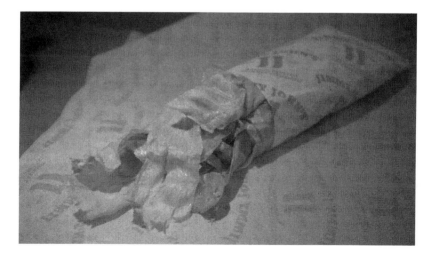

If this is easy for you to do, feel free to eliminate the next item on the list. If you want drastic results, eliminate them all. I have seen one of my client's waistlines shrink inches in just 30 days, but he had only lost five pounds. Why the drastic loss of inches but not a drastic loss in weight? He gave up these inflammatory foods and the swelling simply went down.

THE OMEGA-3 TO OMEGA-6 RATIO

This is a very confusing topic and I have yet to master understanding it but I want to pass on what I know. The confusing part is the science. There are a lot of acronyms and science-y words that confuse my poor uneducated brain. But, what I can gather is that the consumption of too many omega-6s compared to omega-3s is no bueno. Please note the quote below from PubMed.gov.

"Excessive amounts of omega-6 polyunsaturated fatty acids (PUFA) and a very high omega-6/omega-3 ratio, as is found in today's Western diets, promote the pathogenesis of many diseases, including cardiovascular disease, cancer, and inflammatory and autoimmune diseases, whereas increased levels of omega-3 PUFA (a low omega-6/omega-3 ratio) exert suppressive effects."

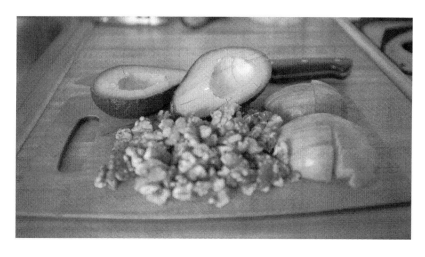

What most people don't know is that we, as Americans, are eating too many foods high in omega-6. Omega-6 is found in commercially raised and grain fed animals. Beef, pork, chicken and fish that is not wild caught or pastured is throwing off your Omega-6 to Omega-3 ratio. This is nothing compared to the amount of omega-6 you get from industrial seed and vegetable oil! Notice the bottom five oils on the list below. They happen to also be the most commonly used oils for frying.

Type of oil	Omega-3	Omega-6
Flaxseed oil	57	16
Rapeseed oil	10	22
Soybean oil	7	54
Walnut oil	5	51
Olive oil	1	8
Corn oil	1	61
Peanut oil	0	33
Safflower oil	0	77
Sesame oil	0	41
Sunflower oil	0	69

Source: U.S. Department of Agriculture

So let's take a look at one of Americas favorite meal, burger and fries. The beef is inflammatory and high in omega-6, the oil the fries are cooked in is inflammatory and high in omega-6, and don't forget the bun itself is a source of inflammation (wheat). This is why so many of us are fat and why even more of us are sick. One thing that sticks out to me is how good people feel when the start a juice cleanse or a vegetarian diet. They are, by default, drastically eliminating the amount of omega-6 they are consuming. Personally, I knew fried foods were bad for you but I thought it was because of the wheat in the batter or breading. This breaks my heart because I love french fries.

Besides eliminating fried foods, what is the best way to improve out omega-6/omega-3 ratio? By simply replacing the animal fat you consume— that's high omega-6, with those high in omega-3.

This is done my eating pasture raised or wild caught meat, fish, fowl, and eggs. Yes, replacing farm-raised salmon with wild caught salmon means you are consuming fats high in omega-3 rather than omega-6. How can the same animal produce difference qualities of fat? Simple, one is fed GRAIN.

Action Step: Stop consuming vegetable oils. If you are going to cook in oil, use coconut oil. If you want to use oil as or for a salad dressing use olive oil. These are the only exceptions.

Also, start using butter from grass fed cows. Number one brand I know of is Kerrygold. I have even seen it in the commissary. It's guilt free butter and will actually help reduce your waist circumference.

WEIGHT LOSS, EXERCISE

You probably don't want to hear this, but if you are not passing the waist measurement part of the PT Test, you are probably overweight. I know, I know. You can do your job. You are in better shape than your skinny counterparts. You work out on a regular basis. The waist measurement is a terrible way to gauge if someone is fit. You're tall (This one has no merit at all). The Air Force just wants Airmen who look good in uniform. Did I miss any? These are not only excuses I have heard; they are excuses I have made. Excuses I made when I had a 40-inch waist. Now, in hindsight and with a 36-inch waist, I see that I was just fat.

This is, no doubt, a tough topic to cover. I cover it in depth in my book, Stop Working Out! And 17 other crazy weight loss tips that actually work. There are many directions we can go with this so I will take the next few chapters to cover as many as I can. Weight loss should be natural and effortless. If you have to try to lose or maintain a weight, you are doing something wrong. For example, if you ever "got fat" because you went on vacation and didn't work out for two weeks, you are doing something wrong. You shouldn't have to rely on something external to maintain your body composition. This leads perfectly into the first part of this topic.

"Excess exercise tends to be counterbalanced by excess hunger, exemplified by the phrase 'working up an appetite.' A few people with extraordinary willpower can resist such hunger day after day, but for the vast majority, weight loss through exercise is a flawed option." ~Andrew Weil M.D.

The first thing I want to do is quash the old standard that is commonly said by people who are not overweight, "Eat less; exercise more." It's crap and doesn't work. Being overweight is not a math problem. It's a chemistry problem, which is a lot harder to figure out. If you think eating less and exercising more works, go for it. But I have to ask, how is it working for you so far? In fact, how is it working for the rest of America? Have you been to a gym lately? It's full of overweight people. You don't think it's their first day, do you?

Ben Davis is the founder of the Do Life movement, motivational speaker, and author of "Do Life." Ben was morbidly obese and decided to start running one day and as a result, he lost 120 pounds. I was very impressed by Ben and started following his blog in 2011. Eventually, I noticed that Ben started posting pictures of his scale. He mentioned how he was gaining weight and needed to get back on track. He was very public about his quest to lose the weight he had gained. Then he disappeared for a while. He came back though, with another picture of the scale and another declaration that he was going to get back on track. This process repeated for the next three years. With each picture of the scale the number showing his weight got higher and higher. Ben actually now weighs more than he did when he started his 120-pound weight loss journey. (I just tried to verify this by checking his website but it appears he has taken down ALL the scale pictures. Including the most recent which showed what he is currently weighing.)

There are many more examples like this out there. Many of the contestants of The Biggest Loser have gained weight since leaving the show. Maybe you know someone who started working out and lost a bunch of weight only to gain it all back. My point is, exercise has very little to do with weight loss. It comes down to a lot more than burning more calories than you consume. It has to do with hormones, habits and your subconscious mind. This may cause you to ask yourself, why do we exercise, then? Well, it's to strengthen. Strengthen your muscles, heart, lungs, circulatory system, bones, and everything else. If nothing else, as Airmen, we exercise so that we can meet the standards of our physical fitness assessment.

Action Step: Change the reason why you are "working out" or "training."

Personally, I am training to get the highest score I've ever gotten on my next PT Test. The last PT test of my career. What are you training for? (This was my reason for training at the time I wrote this. I achieved my goal and retired with the highest score of my career, a 97.5.)

WEIGHT LOSS, KETO

One of the most effective ways to lose weight, specifically fat, is a Ketogenic Diet.

A ketogenic diet, keto for short, is also known as a low carb diet. Keto is most commonly associated with Dr. Robert Atkins, as it is the introductory phase of his diet plan that became popular in the late 90s. Dr. Atkins originally published his book, Dr. Atkins Diet Revolution, in 1972. You would think that this makes him one of the pioneers of keto but, come to find out, he was nearly 200 years behind. John Rollo M.D. was a Scottish military surgeon who treated an army officer for Type II diabetes with a ketogenic diet in 1797.

So what does Type II diabetes have to do with being overweight? We'll get to that in a minute. First, lets clarify what keto actually is.

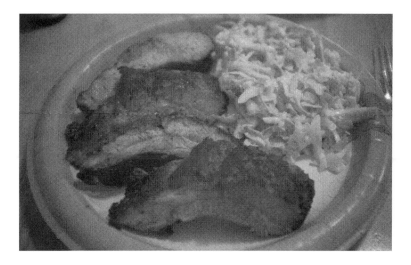

A ketogenic diet is when your food consumption consists of mainly fat. You restrict your carbohydrate intake and moderate your protein consumption to a point that your body goes into ketosis. Ketosis is when your body starts to use fat for energy instead of sugar. Once in this state, if you are overweight, your body will start burning your stored fat for energy, resulting in weight loss. Simple, right?

Let's dig a little deeper and look at how we get overweight in the first place. Our body keeps sugar on hand for energy use in the form of glycogen. Glycogen is stored in your liver and your muscles. When it's needed, like for your super cool crossfit workout, these stores are depleted. If these stores are full when you eat something sugary or starchy (which turns to sugar), like most of the things in your squadron's break-room, then insulin will carry the sugar to fat cells, saving it for later. This is how we get fat.

When you eat a doughnut, the sugar and the flour cause your blood sugar levels with spike, almost immediately. This signals your pancreas to release insulin so it can do its job, which is to regulate your blood sugar levels by delivering the sugar to your muscles and liver in the form of glycogen. Again, if these glycogen stores are full, the insulin carries the sugar to fat cells for storage making the fat cells larger. If you eat another doughnut, or wash it down with a latte, this process continues. Taxing your pancreas like this may not be so bad on occasion but if it happens everyday, meal after meal, you are going to develop problems.

Problem 1: Your liver and muscles no longer respond to the insulin. They become resistant and tell insulin to bugger off. This is known as "Insulin Resistance" and can be an indicator of, or lead to, pre-diabetes.

Problem 2: Your pancreas says, screw it. After years of trying to regulate your blood sugar, your pancreas will eventually just call it quits. When this happens, congratulations, you're diabetic.

Problem 3: High blood sugar, which can affect anything that relies on blood flow in order to work. These are some of the best parts of your body. These include your eyes, your kidneys, your heart, your feet, and your brain. Oh, and the male reproductive organ. (Actually, constant high blood sugar affects your entire body. What I listed are the most common problem areas diabetics suffer difficulties in.)

So why all this high blood sugar, diabetes talk? Well, I'm trying to make something very clear. If your glycogen stores are full or are resistant, insulin will carry blood sugar to your fat cells to be stored, making you fat. The more insulin released into your blood, the more sugar it will take to your fat cells, making you fatter. When is insulin released in to your blood? As soon as you eat something with sugar, or something that turns to sugar, like flour. In the example of the doughnut I have been using, it's sort of a double whammy. Also, keep in mind that insulin is released every time you eat protein too, just not as extreme as with flour and sugar. This kills TWO major weight loss theories: 1) Eat lean proteins and 2) eat small meals throughout the day. Both of these release insulin in your blood and if there is insulin in your blood, you WILL NOT burn stored fat. In fact, the exact opposite happens.

Now we can go back to the question, what does Type II diabetes have to do with being overweight? The answer is that they are both caused by the same thing— the over-consumption of carbohydrates— and a ketogenic diet can reverse them both! You can't address one without addressing the other.

WEIGHT LOSS, KETO FAQS

Ok, you convinced me to go keto so, how do I go about doing it?

This is pretty simple, lower your carb intake. This is done by avoiding starchy carbs like, rice, pasta, breads, potatoes, etc. Some people like to put a number on it like, no more than 20 grams of carbs a day. This is not a bad way to go but I am a fan of simplicity so, I went the unweighed an unmeasured method and stuck with only eating meat, fish, fowl, seeds, nuts, good fats, and low glycemic vegetables (greens mainly).

What are good fats?

Easy answer: Animal fat like lard and tallow, butter, avocados, coconut oil, and olive oil.

Fats to avoid: Soybean oil, canola oil, corn oil, industrial seed oils and, if possible, animal fat from conventionally (not pastured and not grass fed) raised cattle. To understand why this is important, go back to the chapter on the Omega 3 - Omega 6 ratio.

What about dairy?

If you go the Atkins's route, dairy is ok but remember we are trying to pass our PT Test and, for some of us, this means losing inches off our waist. If you recall we can shrink our waist by reducing inflammation. So, dairy should be avoided because of the inflammatory response it causes. Plus dairy has lactose in it, which is a carb.

What about training?

This is probably the most important question of them all. If you are looking to improve your run time, going keto is not going to work for you. Intense training requires glycogen. If you are in ketosis, once you use up all your glycogen stores, they will not get refilled. This will cause you to hit a wall in your training sessions. The energy to train just won't be there. This doesn't mean you can't be active. You just can expect to excel at high intensity, glycogen-demanding workouts.

A good rule of thumb for training while on keto is, subtract your age from 180 and try to keep your heart rate under this number but this won't really help you with improving your mile and half time, not if it's coming up soon. So, you have to pick your battle: Lose Weight or Train.

Personally, once I got my mile and half down to a respectable time, I went keto to slim down. While leaning out, I maintained my endurance by doing low intensity runs until test day.

Do I have to eat this way forever?

Depends, if you are highly sensitive or addicted to sugar, it might be a good idea. Alcoholics don't have cheat days or reintroduce booze after a short period of time. If sugar is your booze, you may want to consider never going back.

However, many people have great success with what is called a Cyclical Ketogenic diet. This is where you are keto 5 to 6 days a week in any combination of days on and days off. This is very handy for people who like to do some intense training a couple days a week.

I recommend staying keto until you hit your goal weight. Once you hit your goal weight (Meaning: repaired your metabolic syndrome), you should be able to reintroduce some carbs back into your diet. Keep in mind this means fruits, squashes, root vegetables, and tubers NOT bagels and donuts. If you went keto to lose weight, hit your goal, and then go back to how you were eating before, you will gain all the weight back.

Can I pig out as long as I don't eat carbs?

Not really. In most cases you will feel very satisfied with your meals and, if you listen to your body, you will stop eating once you are full. There are some exceptions and those are called hyper palatable foods. These are foods that you just enjoy eating and can eat until they are gone. For me, these come in the for of macadamia nuts or pistachios. They are crunchy and delicious and I love them!

Just like anything else, even in a high fat diet, there is a line where you can over do it. Keep this in mind when you are shoving slices of meatzza in your face.

WEIGHT LOSS, OVEREATING

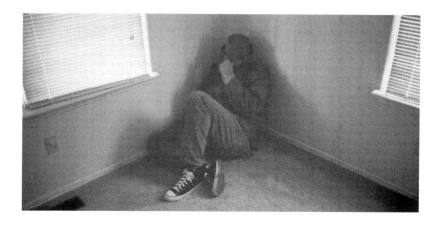

Let's face it, if you are overweight it's because you're overeating. You are overeating because something is bothering you and eating makes you feel better. Trust me, I've been there.

Constant, unnecessary, emotional stress has several negative effects on our body. The least of which is causing us to get fat. Dr. John Sarno, author of Healing Back Pain: The Mind-Body Connection, claims that the majority of back pain is psychosomatic. It is a distraction. Your body creates this pain to distract you from what is really bothering you.

What Dr. Sarno did with his patients was examine them to make sure that something physically wasn't wrong. If he found that there was nothing physically wrong with his patient, he would tell them that it's due to something that was bothering them, that their back pain was emotional. Many people would get instant relief upon simply just hearing this and would walk out of his office feeling better. This happened so much that he started to address entire crowds of patients at once, curing many people of their back problems with a lecture.

My point here is to make you aware that emotional stress can very much, have a physical impact on your body.

It's important to note that Dr. Sarno's patients didn't fix their emotional issues; they simply identified what was bothering them. I think that if we do the same thing here it may be a good jump-start on getting some weight loss results.

I want you to identify what's bothering you. Are you in debt? Does your job suck? What are your living conditions? Anything that is causing you a bunch of stress, I want you to identify it and try to get it out of your life. Like I said, identifying it could be enough. Let's say for example you're $100,000 in debt and it's bothering you. Starting a process to get out of debt may be enough to make you feel better and to jump start your weight loss. You don't have to think that you're going to be overweight until you get your student loans paid off. I'm telling you that just identifying that this is what's bothering you, may be enough to get the weight to start to come off.

Action Step: Identify what's bothering you.

Get piece of paper and a pen out and write this as a header, "Things that are bothering me." Then, underneath start a list of things in your life that are causing you unnecessary emotional stress. That's your first step. Next up, take action and try to remedy each one. But, like I said, identifying them maybe enough. There may be some items that will require you to dig deep. Remember, it's ok to get some help.

YES, THAT'S REALLY IT.

I am a minimalist in everything I do, to include how I write. I get straight to the point and, curiously, I found many people appreciate that. So yeah, that's it!

Please, please, please feel free to contact me if you need any help. I will be more than happy to answer any questions you have or even do a free coaching call. I have noticed an upswing in book sales and I personally want to thank every person who has read this book.

If you like what you just read, please check out my other books on amazon and please leave a review for this one while you are there. It will really help spread the word. If you didn't like it, however never mind. ;-)

Best of luck,

David Soto Jr, MSgt, USAF (Retired)
Twitter: @davidesotojr
Instagram: @davidesotojr
Website: www.davidsotowrites.com

ABOUT THE AUTHOR

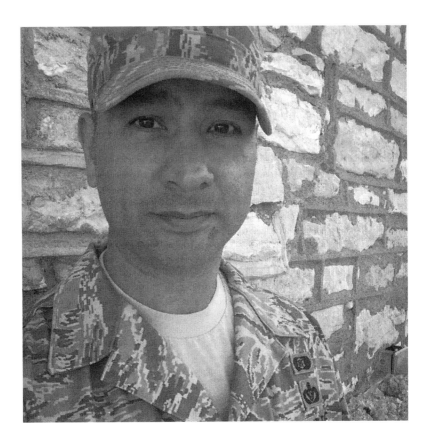

David was born in Gardena, California and spent most of his childhood in Los Angeles. In high school, his family moved to a small town in Missouri. At age 17, David joined the Air Force and spent the next 23 years toggling between active duty Air Force and the Missouri Air National Guard. In 2002 he was deployed under Operation Enduring Freedom and in 2004 he served his country, as a civilian contractor, in Iraq.

Throughout the years, when not in uniform, David tried his best to fit into society. He got a job, went into debt to buy a house and a car, and tried to find a girl to marry and start a family with. None of these seemed to work out for him. Instead, he felt best on the road. At the age of 30, he sold most of his possessions, put his house up for rent, hit the road, and (more or less) hasn't stopped since.

Currently, David is probably somewhere in Colorado trying to catch a trout or in a coffee shop working on his next book.

Made in the USA
Middletown, DE
04 September 2019